how my body works

staying healthy

Barrie Knowles

Wayland

how my body works

Breathing
Eating
Growing
Moving
Sleeping
Staying Healthy

Editor: Anna Girling
Designer: Jean Wheeler

First published in 1992 by
Wayland (Publishers) Ltd
61 Western Road, Hove
East Sussex BN3 1JD, England

British Library Cataloguing in Publication Data
Knowles, Barrie
Staying Healthy. – (How My Body Works Series)
I. Title   II. Series
613

ISBN 0 7502 0434 6

Typeset by Dorchester Typesetting Group Ltd
Printed and bound in Belgium by Casterman S.A.

All words printed in **bold** are explained in the glossary.

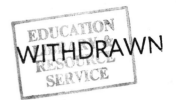

Contents

Am I healthy?

Look at these pictures. Do you think that all these people are healthy?

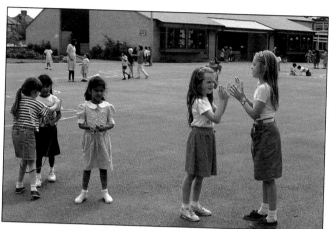

What do you think a healthy person looks like? Draw a picture showing your ideas.

What do you think **health** means?

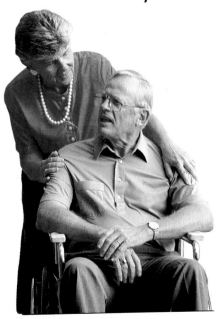

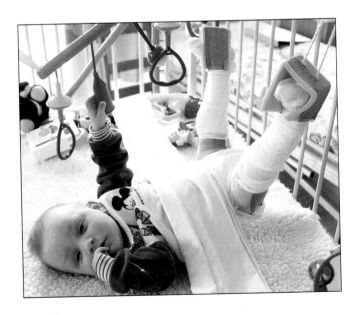

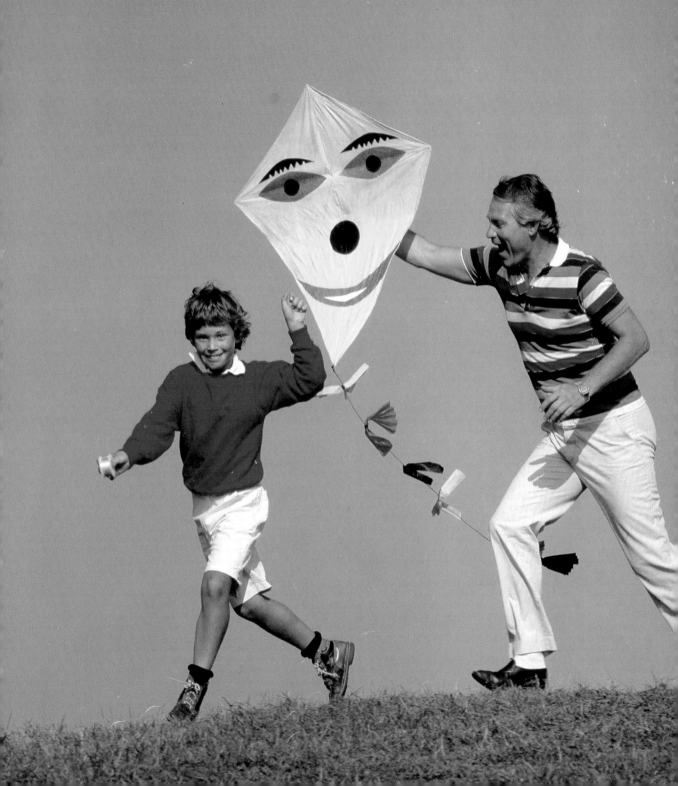

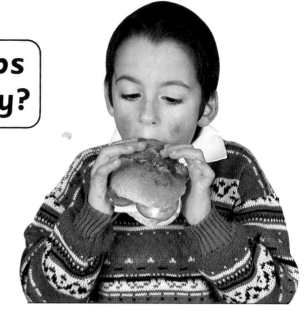

What keeps me healthy?

Food gives you **energy** to stay alive and help your body grow.

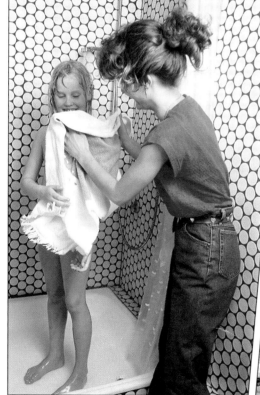

Keeping clean helps you to stay healthy.

You sleep to give your body a rest.

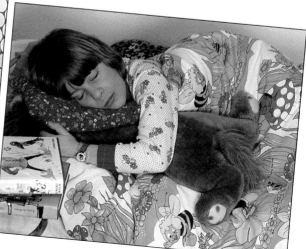

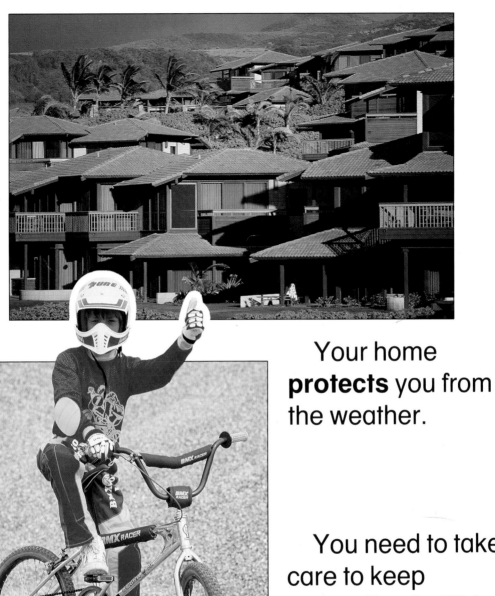

Your home **protects** you from the weather.

You need to take care to keep yourself safe. This cyclist is wearing special clothing to keep himself safe.

What food should I eat?

You have to eat to stay alive. Food gives you energy. Food helps you grow. Some kinds of food help your teeth and bones grow stronger.

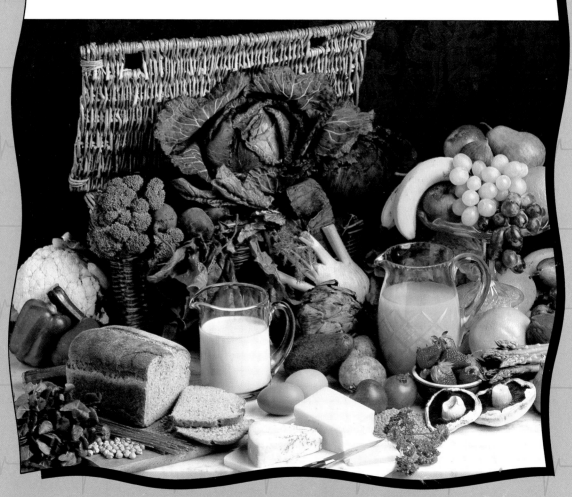

To stay healthy you need to eat a mixture of different kinds of food: fresh fruit and vegetables, bread and **cereals**, milk and cheese, meat and fish.

One of these boys is eating sweets. The other is eating fruit. Which of these foods is better for you?

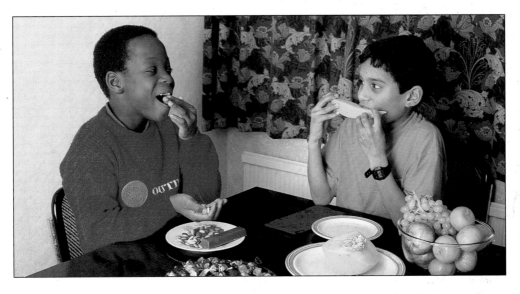

Try to eat foods which do not have much sugar or fat in them.

Too much sugar is bad for your teeth. What can happen if you eat too much fat?

9

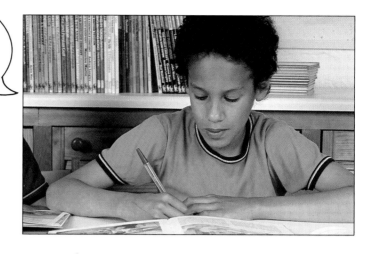

How do I spend my time?

Think of all the things you did yesterday.

This boy is doing school work. How much time did you spend working at school or at home? How much time did you spend asleep?

Did you spend time doing these things?

Reading

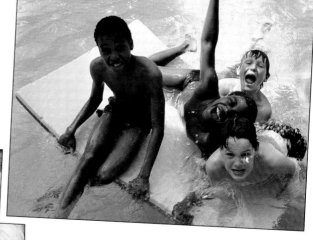

Playing

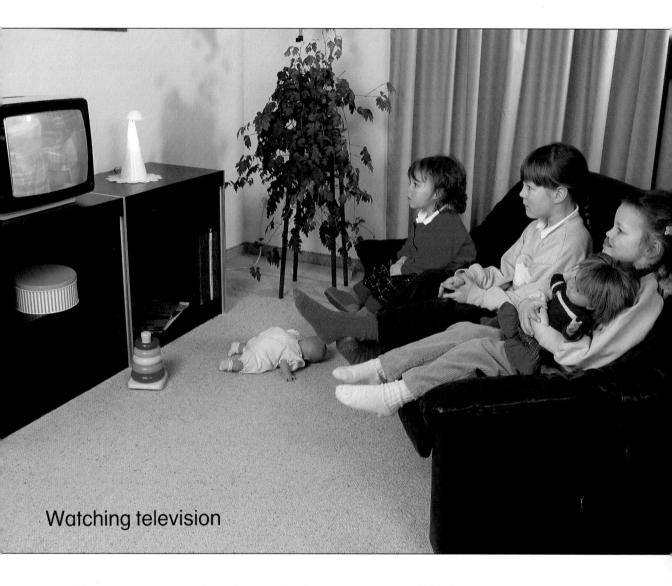

Watching television

If you spend a lot of time **exercising** you get tired and need to rest. Your body needs a chance to recover. Rest and sleep are very important.

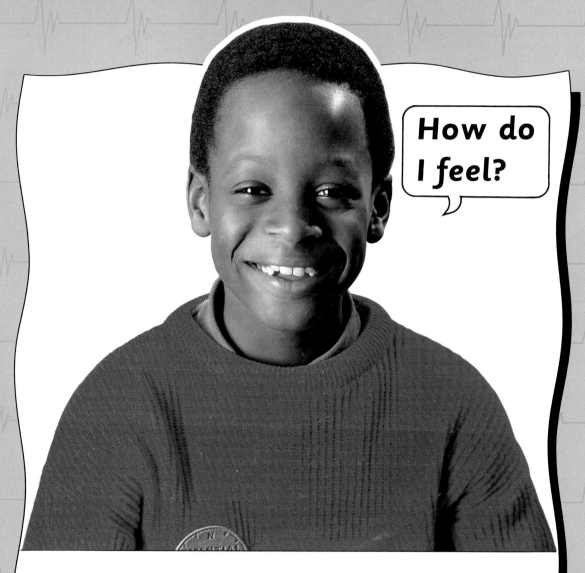

How do I feel?

You can often tell how people feel by the way they look.

These three pictures show a boy when he is happy, sad and surprised. Can you say which one is which?

What sort of things make you happy? Do they always make you happy?

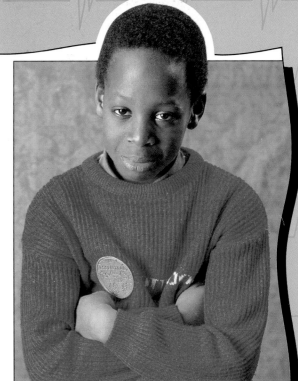

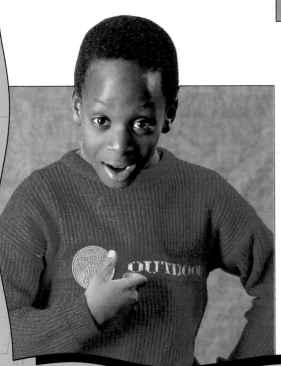

Sometimes it is nice to be with friends. At other times you might like to be on your own.

Why do I need to keep clean?

Keeping healthy through keeping clean is called hygiene.

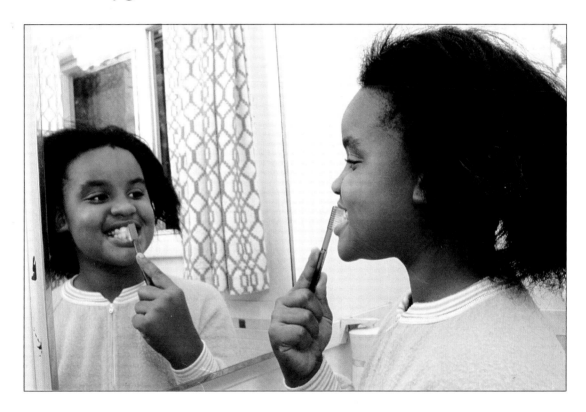

How often do you clean your teeth? Brushing gets rid of any food that is stuck to your teeth. Keeping your teeth clean helps to make them strong and healthy.

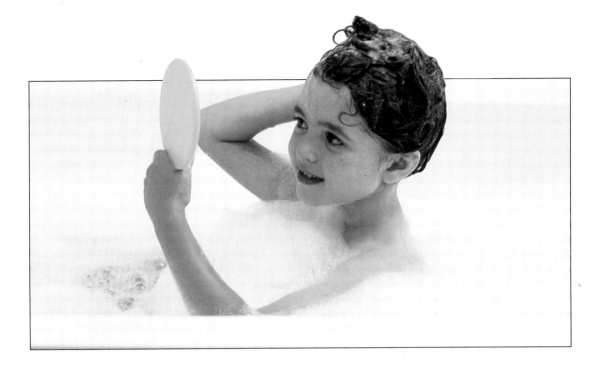

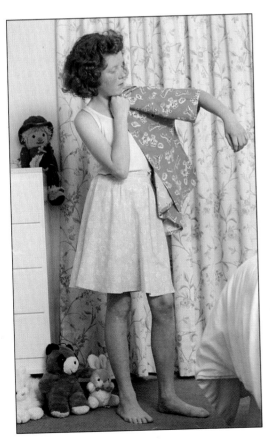

Washing and brushing your hair makes it look good and feel good.

It is important to have a bath or shower regularly. This keeps your skin clean. It makes you smell nice.

Your clothes get dirty too. They also need to be washed often.

What do I use to wash?

What do you use when you
wash your hands?

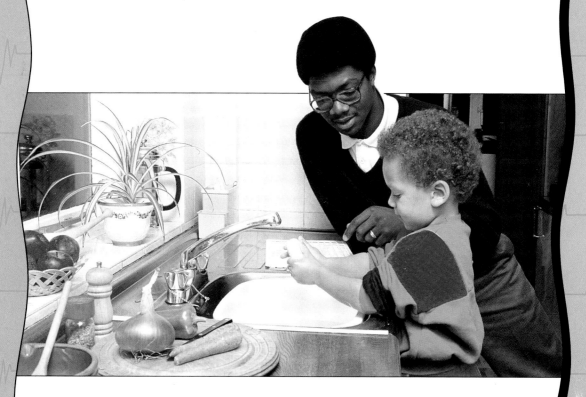

Try the experiment opposite. You will
need some friends to help you. Which of
the four suggestions do you think will work
the best?

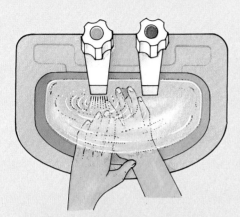

Cold water only

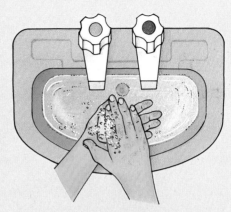

Cold water and soap

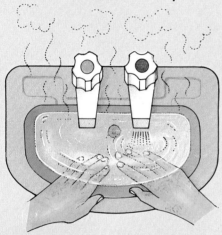

Warm water only

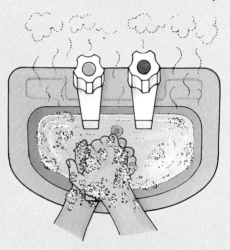

Warm water and soap

What worked best? Were you right with your guess?

What is wrong with this kitchen?

Look at this picture of a kitchen. How many things can you see that make it unhealthy? What would you have to do to make it clean and safe?

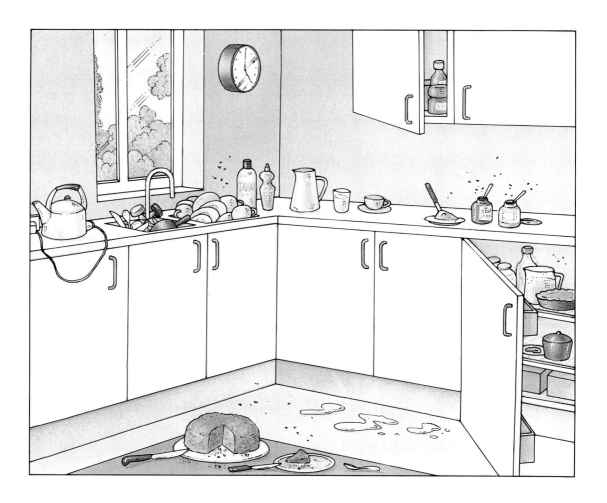

Answers on page 31

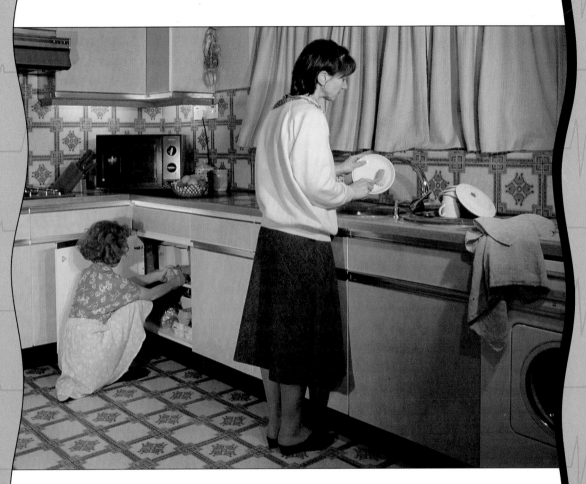

Pots, pans and plates must be washed and put away after they have been used. It is important to keep food covered. It must be kept away from animals and insects.

How do I keep safe?

You need to take care to stay out of danger and keep yourself safe. If you are careful you will have fewer accidents.

In your home there are many things that can hurt you. Electricity, plugs and sockets are very dangerous. You must never play with them.

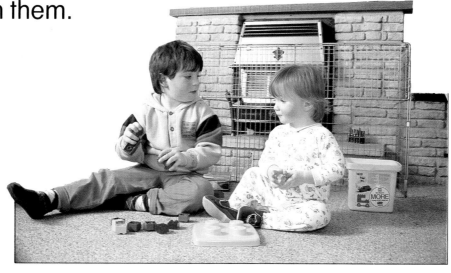

Fires and cookers get very hot. They can burn you. This fire has a guard in front of it to stop the children getting too close.

What else in your home can be dangerous?

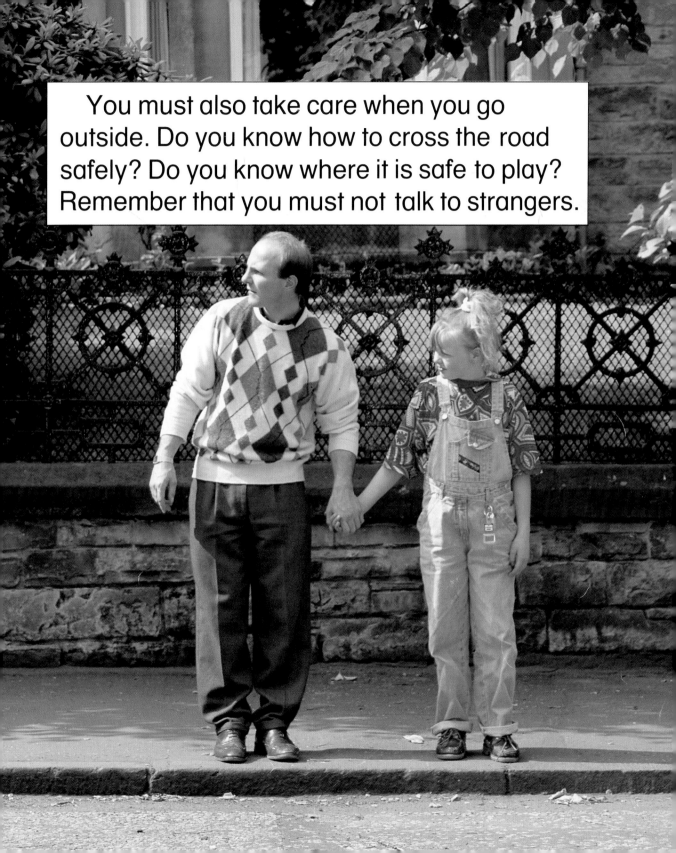

You must also take care when you go outside. Do you know how to cross the road safely? Do you know where it is safe to play? Remember that you must not talk to strangers.

Where is a healthy place to play?

Look at these pictures of playgrounds. How are they different? Which one do you like best?

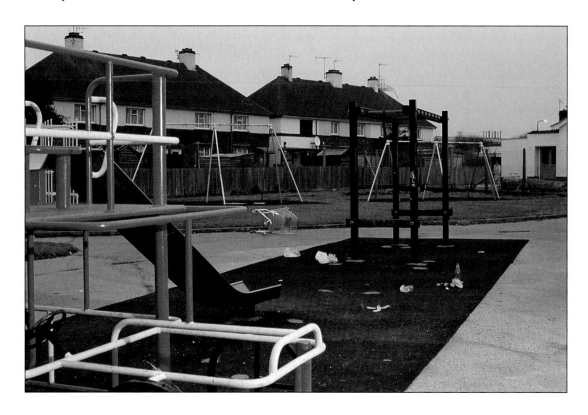

In this playground people have dropped **litter** and left bottles on the ground. Somebody has left an old shopping trolley. Do you think it is wrong to drop litter?

This playground has a safety barrier all round. The ground is soft to fall on. There are grown-ups watching the children playing.

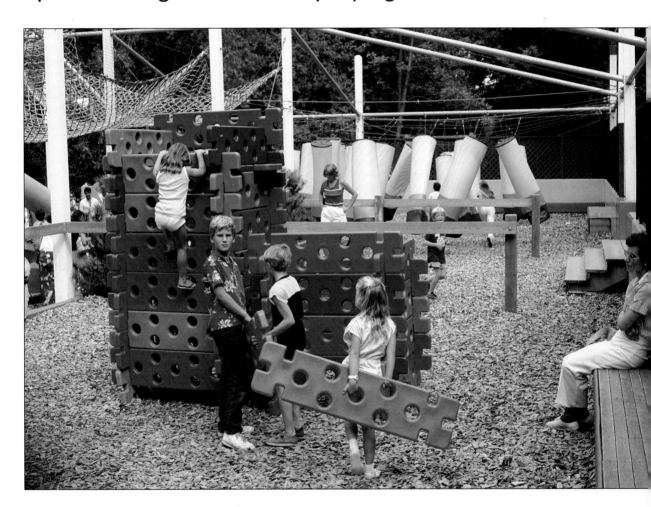

Design a safe playground that you would like to use yourself.

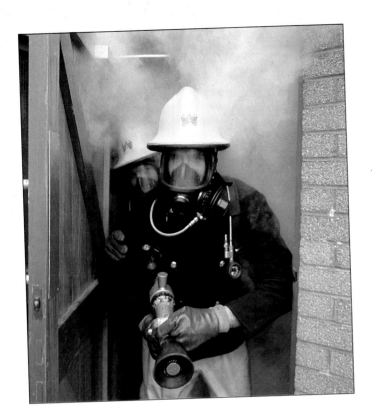

What would you wear?

Some people need to wear special clothing to work.

Firefighters need masks and thick clothes to protect them from smoke and heat.

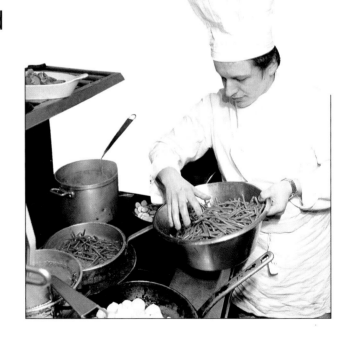

Cooks wear aprons and cover their hair with hats.

This man is wearing a face mask. It protects his eyes and stops him breathing in dust.

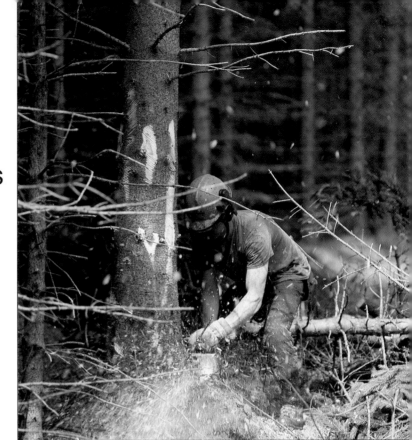

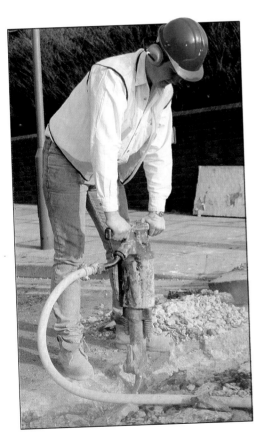

Loud noises can damage your hearing. This man is wearing ear protectors.

We wear different clothes at different times of the year. What do you wear in winter? What do you wear in summer?

Who helps me stay healthy?

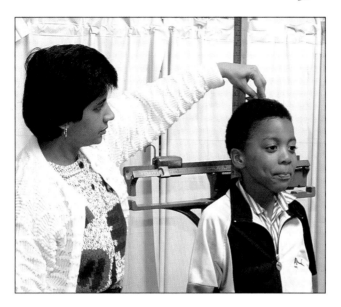

These people help you stay healthy.

A nurse checks your height and weight.

A teacher helps you cross the road.

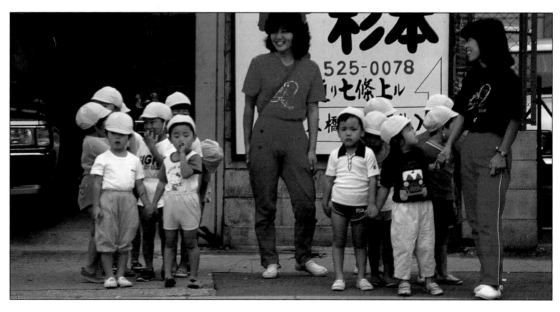

Parents make sure you are safe.
A doctor helps to keep you well.

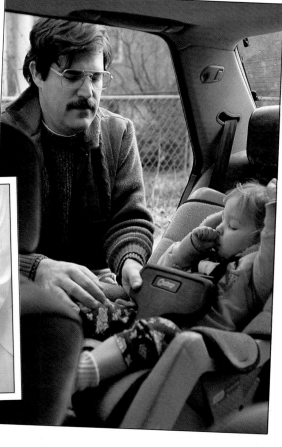

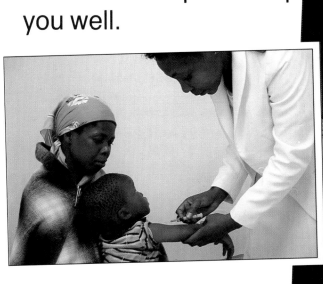

A dentist looks after your teeth.

Can you think of anyone else who helps you?

How can we help other people?

In some parts of the world there is not enough food for everybody. There are many people who are always hungry.

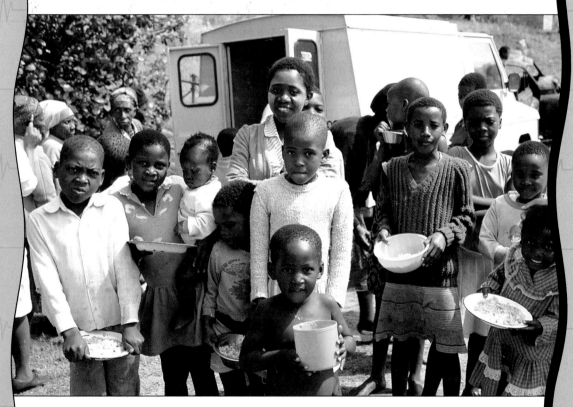

Sometimes they have no clean water to drink. Dirty water causes illnesses.

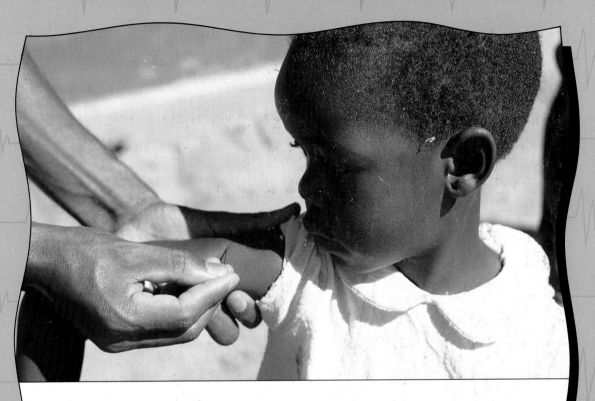

These people need **medicines** to stop illnesses spreading. Some of them do not have a home to live in.

How can you help these people? There are many **charities** that care for people like this. They give food and medicines. They show people how to stay healthy. How can you help these charities to give this special care?

Glossary

Cereals Foods made from corn.
Charities Organizations set up to help other people.
Design Draw a plan for something.
Energy The strength to move and do things.
Exercising Using your muscles and moving about.

Health The state your body and mind are in. If you are in good health you feel well, not ill.
Litter Rubbish that is left lying around.
Medicines Substances that a sick person swallows or puts on their body to make them better.
Protects Keeps safe.

Books to read

Freckly Feet and Itchy Knees by Michael Rosen (Harper Collins, 1990)
Going to the Dentist by Kate Petty and Lisa Kopper (Franklin Watts, 1988)
Going to the Hospital by A. Civardi and S. Cartwright (Usborne, 1986)
The Tale of Mucky Mabel by Jeanne Willis and Margaret Chamberlain (Arrow Books, 1984)
What happens when you catch a cold? by Joy Richardson (Hamish Hamilton, 1984)

Notes on the National Curriculum

This book is relevant to the following Attainment Targets:

	Level	Statements of Attainment
SCIENCE Attainment Target 1: Scientific investigation	1	*Pupils should:* carry out investigations in which they: (a) observe familiar materials and events.
	2	(a) ask questions such as 'how . . . ?', 'why . . . ?' and 'what will happen if . . . ?', suggest ideas and make predictions. (c) use their observations to support conclusions and compare what they have observed with what they expected.
	3	(b) observe closely and quantify by measuring using appropriate instruments.
Attainment Target 2: Life and living processes	2	(a) know that plants and animals need certain conditions to sustain life.
MATHEMATICS Attainment Target 1:	3	*Pupils should:* (c) present results in a clear and organized way.
Attainment Target 2:	1	(a) use number in the context of the classroom and school.
ENGLISH		Children using this book can cover many aspects of the *Reading, Speaking* and *Listening* sections of the National Curriculum.

Answers to page 18

Kettle lead hanging over side; dirty washing up; cleaning liquids left out; food left uncovered; cupboard and refrigerator doors open; dirty floor; flies; knives left out.

Index

Picture acknowledgements

The publishers would like to thank the following: Cephas 25 top; Eye Ubiquitous 15 bottom (Mostyn), 19 (Mostyn), 22 (Mostyn), 25 bottom (Mostyn), 26 bottom (P. Seheult); Chris Fairclough 6 top, 10 top, 24 bottom, 27 bottom; John and Penny Hubley 27 top left, 28; Hutchison Library 29 (S. Errington); PHOTRI 7 top (S. Lissau), 23 (MacDonald), 27 top right; Tony Stone Worldwide cover, 8 (R. Weller); Topham 10 bottom right; Wayland Picture Library 9 (A. Blackburn), 10 bottom left (T. Woodcock), 12 (A. Blackburn), 13 both (A. Blackburn), 16 (T. Hill), 21 (A. Blackburn), 14 top, 26 top (T. Woodcock); Timothy Woodcock 20; Zefa 4 all, 5, 6 bottom left and right, 7 bottom, 11, 14, 15 top. Artwork on pages 17 and 18 by John Yates. Background artwork on pages 8-9, 12-13, 16-17, 19 and 28-9 supplied by Jenny Hughes.